15 FOOD THAT MAKES YOU CONSTIPATED.

Knowing what food to avoid is a necessity.

By

Dr DOUGLAS JASON

TABLE OF CONTENT

ABOUT THE AUTHOR

INTRODUCTION

TABLE OF CONTENTS

ABOUT THE AUTHOR

Dr. Douglas Jason is a certified dietician who has a strong passion for wellness and a big eagerness to help people all over the world. He uses healthy food, herbs, spices, and other useful tools to help mankind realize its overall goal of optimum health.

INTRODUCTION

Constipation is a frequent condition in which people have difficulty passing stools. Medically, constipation is defined as having less than three bowel motions per week.

Severe constipation occurs when a person has fewer than one bowel movement each week. Constipation may be accompanied by symptoms of bloating, gas, or pain during bowel motions.

What foods contribute to constipation?

Numerous foods can help prevent or cure constipation, but some foods can have a binding effect and make your constipation worse. When you're constipated, avoid these 15 foods.

CHAPTER 1

BANANAS

When it comes to constipation foods to avoid, bananas are a riddle. It's all about timing: unripe bananas can promote constipation, while ripe bananas can help cure it.

Unripe or under-ripe green bananas cause constipation because they contain a lot of starch, which the body finds difficult to digest.

Bananas also contain pectin, which pulls water from the intestines into the stool.
If a person is already dehydrated, this can aggravate constipation.

Babies can also become constipated if they consume an excessive amount of bananas. Moderation and a variety of fruits and vegetables for your child are essential.

CHAPTER 2

GUM FOR CHEWING.

It is not true that it takes seven years to digest a piece of gum. However, it is true that swallowing a large amount of gum in a short period, or swallowing multiple pieces of gum with other indigestible items such as seeds, might result in a mass that, in rare situations, stops the digestive tract. Constipation may result from this intestinal obstruction.

Children under the age of five should not chew gum at all, and if you do chew gum, limit yourself to one or two pieces per day – and throw it away when you're through.

CHAPTER 3

CAFFEINE

Caffeine, like bananas, may go either way.

Caffeine is a stimulant that can cause an increase in bowel movements or, in extreme cases, diarrhea.
Caffeine in coffee, black tea, colas, and chocolate can aggravate constipation if a person is dehydrated.

CHAPTER 4

GLUTEN

Gluten is a protein found in grains such as wheat, rye, and barley.
Gluten does not cause constipation in everyone, but it can be an issue for those who are sensitive to it, have allergies to it, or have celiac disease, an autoimmune ailment.

Celiac disease patients must avoid any gluten-containing goods.

Consult your doctor if you suspect you have non-celiac gluten sensitivity, which may be causing your constipation. There are several gluten-free foods available to replace bread and pasta, which often contain gluten.

A bowl of white rice accompanied by chopsticks. Because the husk, bran, and germ have been removed from white rice, it might cause constipation. That is where all of the fiber and nutrients are located!

CHAPTER 5

RICE WHITE

Constipation can be caused by white rice. There is a significant distinction between white rice and brown rice.

Because the husk, bran, and germ have been removed from white rice, it might cause constipation. That is where all of the fiber and nutrients are located!

Because the husk, bran, and germ have not been removed, brown rice can help reduce constipation.

1 cup of brown rice includes about 3.5 g of fiber and 5 g of protein, making it a rich source of whole grains.

CHAPTER 6

PERSIMMON

Persimmon is a fruit that is popular in Asia but is less well-known in the United States. Sweet persimmons are normally fine, but more astringent persimmons contain a lot of tannins, which might slow down digestion and cause constipation.
If you must eat persimmons, choose the sweet type.
A raw ribeye steak cut.

Because red meat has more fat, it takes longer for the digestive tract to metabolize.

CHAPTER 7

MEAT IN RED

There are numerous reasons to avoid eating red meat. Red meat has the potential to cause constipation for a variety of reasons. Red meat:

Because it is high in fat, it takes longer for the digestive tract to process.
Has stiff protein fibers that can be difficult to digest in the stomach

It is high in iron, which can cause constipation.
To avoid constipation, limit your consumption of red meat.

CHAPTER 8

WHITE FLOUR

While whole-grain bread may aid in constipation relief, white bread may induce or worsen it. This also applies to items containing a lot of white flour, such as

bagels,
crackers
pretzels.
White flour, unlike whole grains, contains no fiber.

These foods are high in starch and can help you. Always choose whole grains.

CHAPTER 9

ALCOHOL.

Alcohol, like caffeine, can contribute to constipation. For instance, alcohol

It dehydrates the body and can impede digestion and irritate the colon, exacerbating constipation symptoms.
Limit your alcohol consumption and replace one alcoholic beverage with a glass of water or even a sports drink (such as

Gatorade or Powerade) in between.

A selection of chocolate bars. Chocolate is not recommended, especially for persons who have irritable bowel syndrome (IBS).

Alcohol dehydrates the body and can irritate the intestines, exacerbating constipation symptoms.

CHAPTER 10

CHOCOLATE

Chocolate is not recommended, especially for persons who have irritable bowel syndrome (IBS).

It is thought that the high-fat content of chocolate slows digestion.
It is thought that this occurs by slowing muscle contractions (peristalsis) and thus slowing

food movement through the gut.

In one study, researchers in Germany asked participants suffering from constipation to name the items they believed were to blame. Chocolate was cited the most.

A table with dairy items such as milk, cheese, yogurt, and butter.

Constipation may be caused by taking iron and calcium supplements.

CHAPTER 11

SOME SUPPLEMENTS ARE.

Many people take iron and calcium supplements to keep healthy, yet these same nutrients may be the cause of constipation. A healthy, balanced diet should ideally offer all of the nutrients a person requires.

If your doctor advises you to take these supplements (for example, persons with anemia require iron, and women at risk of osteoporosis may require calcium), remember to include foods high in fiber in your diet to aid with constipation.

Dairy items in a take-out tray. Dairy items, such as milk, cheese, yogurt, and ice cream, can cause constipation in significant quantities.

CHAPTER 12

DAIRY PRODUCTS ARE DISCUSSED

Dairy items, such as milk, cheese, yogurt, and ice cream, can cause constipation in significant quantities. It could be because of dairy or a combination of factors. The lactose in dairy, on the other hand, might create increased gas and bloating, which can make a person feel even worse if things aren't flowing through properly.

One research of Iranian children aged one to thirteen discovered that dairy products could be the source of their constipation. Almost all of the children (80%) who avoided cow's milk and milk products had more regular bowel movements.

Burgers and fries are heavy in fat and poor in fiber.
Dairy items, such as milk, cheese, yogurt, and ice cream,

can cause constipation in significant quantities.

CHAPTER 13

FAST FOOD

All of those burgers and fries are heavy in fat and poor in fiber. Fried meals might cause constipation. Not to add that quick foods frequently lack nutritional content.

Try these instead of a fast-food burger and fries:

Make your burgers using lean ground turkey, or try a veggie

patty on a whole-grain wheat bun.

Sweet potatoes are high in soluble fiber and minerals, and they can help relieve and prevent constipation. So, instead of regular French fries, try baked sweet potato fries. Leave the skin on since it contains the most fiber!

A frozen turkey, potato, and pea meal.

Dairy items, such as milk, cheese, yogurt, and ice cream, can cause constipation in significant quantities.

CHAPTER 14

PROCESSED FOODS AND FROZEN DINNERS

Processed foods, like fast foods, have little nutrients and frequently a lot of fat. Many of them are also high in salt. Examples of foods to avoid include

White bread, pastries, prepared dinners, chips, and hot dogs are all options.

Constipation can be caused by any of these foods because they slow down the digestive system. Snack on fruits, vegetables, and meals in their natural form, and drink plenty of water to keep your digestive system running smoothly.

A potato chip bag
Potato chips are delicious, but they are heavy in fat (high-fat foods can impede digestion), low in fiber, and deficient in almost every other vitamin.

CHAPTER 15

CHIPPING

Potato chips are delicious, but they are heavy in fat (high-fat foods can impede digestion), low in fiber, and deficient in almost every other vitamin. People frequently aimlessly nibble on chips to fill themselves up.
Instead, nibble on raw vegetables for a delightful crunch from fiber-rich meals.

Top 4 Constipation Relief Foods

Here is a list of four meals that can help you get rid of constipation.

Beans\sBerries\sKiwi\sFlaxseed...

www.ingramcontent.com/pod-product-compliance
Lightning Source LLC
Chambersburg PA
CBHW071113220526
45467CB00004B/1842